The Power of Mindfulness: Using Meditation to Aid in Weight Loss

Contents

Left blank intentionally

CHAPTER ONE

Introduction: The Connection Between Meditation and Weight Loss

The connection between meditation and weight loss is not immediately obvious.

However, when we examine the underlying causes of weight gain, it becomes clear that meditation may be a powerful tool for addressing them.

For many people, weight gain is the result of emotional eating. When we are stressed, anxious, or bored, we often turn to food as a way of coping with our feelings. Unfortunately, this can lead to a cycle of overeating and weight gain.

Meditation can help break this cycle by teaching us to become more aware of our emotions and our relationship with food. By practicing mindfulness, we can learn to recognize when we are feeling stressed or anxious, and we can learn to respond to these feelings in a more productive way.

Another way in which meditation can promote weight loss is by reducing stress levels. When we are stressed, our bodies produce cortisol, a hormone that can increase appetite and promote fat storage. By reducing stress levels, meditation can help to lower cortisol levels and promote weight loss.

In addition to these benefits, meditation can also help to improve our overall relationship with our bodies. When we meditate, we learn to become more aware of our thoughts and feelings, and we can begin to develop a greater sense of self-compassion and self-acceptance.

This can be especially important for people who struggle with body image issues. By learning to accept and love ourselves just as we are, we may be more likely to make healthy choices and to feel motivated to take care of our bodies.

Overall, the connection between meditation and weight loss is complex and multifaceted. While meditation is not a magic bullet for weight loss, it can be a powerful tool for promoting mindfulness, reducing stress levels, and improving our overall relationship with our bodies.

In the following chapters, we will explore the benefits of meditation for weight loss in more detail. We will examine the science behind meditation and weight loss, and we will provide practical tips and strategies for incorporating meditation into your weight loss journey.

By the end of this guide, you will have a better understanding of the connection between meditation and weight loss, and you will have the tools and knowledge you need to start using meditation to achieve your weight loss goals.

CHAPTER TWO

Understanding Meditation: What It Is and How It Works

Meditation is a practice that has been around for thousands of years, with roots in many different cultures and spiritual traditions. Despite its long history, many people are still unsure about what meditation is and how it works.

At its core, meditation is a mental practice that involves focusing your attention on a particular object, thought, or activity. This might be a specific word or phrase (known as a mantra), your breath, or an image in your mind.

The goal of meditation is to cultivate a state of calm, focused awareness. By training your mind to focus on a single point of focus, you can learn to quiet the constant chatter of your thoughts and achieve a sense of inner peace.

While the idea of focusing your mind on a single point might seem simple, it can be quite challenging in practice. Our minds are naturally restless and easily distracted, and it can take time and practice to train ourselves to stay focused.

One of the keys to successful meditation is to approach it with a sense of curiosity and non-judgment. Rather than trying to force your mind to be still or to stop thinking altogether, simply observe your thoughts as they arise and gently redirect your attention back to your point of focus.

Over time, this practice can have profound effects on your mental and physical health. Research has shown that meditation can reduce stress, improve mood, boost immune function, and even change the structure of the brain.

One of the ways that meditation can have such powerful effects on the brain is through a process called neuroplasticity. Neuroplasticity refers to the brain's ability to change and adapt in response to new experiences.

When we meditate, we are essentially rewiring our brains to be calmer and more focused. By consistently directing our attention to a single point, we are strengthening the neural connections associated with focus and attention.

This, in turn, can help to reduce activity in the default mode network (DMN), a network of brain regions that is active when we are not focused on a specific task. The DMN is associated with mind-wandering and self-referential thinking, and it has been linked to anxiety and depression.

By reducing activity in the DMN, meditation can help to quiet the mind and reduce feelings of anxiety and stress. It can also help to improve our ability to regulate our emotions and make better decisions.

While meditation is often associated with spiritual or religious practices, it is important to note that you don't have to be religious to practice meditation. Meditation is simply a mental practice that anyone can do, regardless of their religious or spiritual beliefs.

There are many different types of meditation, each with its own unique focus and approach. Some of the most common types of meditation include mindfulness meditation, loving-kindness meditation, and transcendental meditation.

In the following chapters, we will explore each of these types of meditation in more detail, and we will provide practical tips and strategies for incorporating meditation into your daily life.

By the end of this guide, you will have a better understanding of what meditation is and how it works. You will also have the tools and knowledge you need to start practicing meditation and experiencing the many benefits that it can offer.

CHAPTER THREE

BENEFITS OF MEDITATION FOR WEIGHT LOSS

Meditation is a powerful tool that can be used to promote weight loss and improve overall health and well-being. While it may seem unlikely that sitting quietly and focusing your mind could have any impact on your weight, research has shown that meditation can have a number of positive effects on the body that can lead to weight loss and improved health.

One of the most important ways that meditation can help with weight loss is by reducing stress levels. Stress is a common trigger for overeating and emotional eating, as it can lead to the release of the hormone cortisol, which can increase appetite and cravings for high-calorie foods.

When we meditate, we activate the body's relaxation response, which can help to counteract the effects of stress. By reducing levels of cortisol and other stress hormones, meditation can help to reduce cravings and make it easier to stick to a healthy eating plan.

In addition to reducing stress, meditation can also help to improve sleep quality, which is an important factor in weight loss. Lack of sleep has been linked to weight gain and obesity, as it can disrupt hormones that regulate appetite and metabolism.

By promoting relaxation and reducing stress, meditation can help to improve the quality and duration of sleep, leading to better weight management and improved overall health.

Another way that meditation can aid in weight loss is by promoting mindful eating. Mindful eating involves paying close attention to the experience of eating, including the taste, texture, and smell of the food, as well as the feelings of hunger and fullness.

By practicing mindful eating during meals and snacks, we can become more attuned to our body's hunger and satiety signals, which can help to prevent overeating and improve food choices.

Meditation can also help to improve body awareness and body image, which are important factors in weight loss. By practicing meditation regularly, we can become more attuned to our body's needs and more accepting of our physical appearance, which can reduce feelings of stress and shame related to weight and body image.

Finally, meditation can help to improve overall health and well-being, which can contribute to long-term weight loss success. Regular meditation practice has been linked to improved immune function, reduced inflammation, and better cardiovascular health, among other benefits.

By promoting overall health and well-being, meditation can help to create a positive feedback loop that supports healthy habits and long-term weight management.

In conclusion, meditation is a powerful tool that can be used to support weight loss and improve overall health and well-being. By reducing stress levels, improving sleep quality, promoting mindful eating, and improving body awareness and acceptance, meditation can help to create a positive and sustainable approach to weight management.

If you are interested in incorporating meditation into your weight loss journey, start by setting aside just a few minutes each day to practice. Find a quiet and comfortable place to sit, close your eyes, and focus your attention on your breath or a specific object or mantra.

Over time, you may find that meditation becomes a natural and enjoyable part of your daily routine, and that it helps to support your weight loss goals and overall health and well-being.

CHAPTER FOUR

Science Behind Meditation: How It Affects the Brain and Body

Meditation has become a popular practice in recent years for reducing stress and promoting relaxation. However, the benefits of meditation go beyond just mental and emotional well-being. Scientific research has shown that meditation can also have a profound impact on the body, including weight loss.

One of the key ways that meditation affects the body is through its impact on the brain. When we meditate, we enter a state of deep relaxation that can help to reduce stress and anxiety. This, in turn, helps to reduce the production of the stress hormone cortisol, which has been linked to weight gain and difficulty losing weight.

Meditation has also been shown to have a positive effect on the digestive system. When we are stressed, our digestive system shuts down, making it more difficult to digest food and absorb nutrients. This can lead to weight gain and other digestive problems. By reducing stress and promoting relaxation, meditation can help to improve digestion and promote healthy weight loss.

In addition to its effects on the brain and digestive system, meditation has also been shown to have a positive impact on the immune system. Research has shown that regular meditation can help to strengthen the immune system, which can help to ward off illnesses and prevent weight gain caused by illness.

Another way that meditation can help with weight loss is by promoting healthy habits. When we meditate, we become more aware of our thoughts and emotions. This heightened awareness can help us to identify unhealthy habits and patterns, such as emotional eating or mindless snacking. By becoming more mindful of our actions, we can make more conscious decisions about what we eat and how we live, which can help to support healthy weight loss.

Finally, meditation can help to promote overall well-being, which is essential for healthy weight loss. When we are stressed or anxious, we are more likely to turn to food for comfort. By promoting relaxation and reducing stress, meditation can help to break the cycle of emotional eating and support healthy weight loss.

Overall, the science behind meditation and its impact on the body is complex and multifaceted. However, the benefits of meditation for weight loss are clear. By reducing stress, promoting healthy habits, and supporting overall well-being, meditation can be a powerful tool for those looking to lose weight and improve their health.

CHAPTER FIVE

Types of Meditation: Which Ones Are Best for Weight Loss

Meditation is a practice that has been used for centuries to promote relaxation, reduce stress, and improve overall well-being. However, not all types of meditation are created equal when it comes to weight loss. Different types of meditation can have different effects on the body and mind, making some more effective than others for promoting healthy weight loss. In this article, we will explore some of the different types of meditation and discuss which ones are best for weight loss.

Mindfulness Meditation

Mindfulness meditation is a type of meditation that involves focusing on the present moment and being fully aware of one's thoughts and feelings without judgment. It has been shown to be effective for reducing stress and anxiety, improving emotional well-being, and promoting healthy eating habits. By becoming more mindful of our thoughts and emotions, we can identify unhealthy patterns and behaviors that may be contributing to weight gain.

Loving-Kindness Meditation

Loving-kindness meditation is a type of meditation that involves cultivating feelings of love, compassion, and kindness towards oneself and others. It has been shown to be effective for reducing stress, improving emotional well-being, and promoting healthy relationships. By cultivating feelings of self-love and compassion, we can improve our relationship with food and develop a more positive body image.

Transcendental Meditation

Transcendental meditation is a type of meditation that involves using a mantra or sound to focus the mind and achieve a deep state of relaxation. It has been shown to be effective for reducing stress, improving emotional well-being, and promoting overall health. By achieving a state of deep relaxation, we can reduce the production of the stress hormone cortisol, which can contribute to weight gain.

Yoga

Yoga is a type of meditation that involves physical movement and breathwork. It has been shown to be effective for reducing stress, improving flexibility and balance, and promoting overall health. By practicing yoga, we can improve our physical health and reduce stress, which can contribute to healthy weight loss.

Body Scan Meditation

Body scan meditation is a type of meditation that involves focusing on different parts of the body and becoming aware of any physical sensations or tension. It has been shown to be effective for reducing stress, improving sleep, and promoting overall health. By becoming more aware of our physical sensations, we can identify areas of tension and stress that may be contributing to weight gain.

In conclusion, there are many different types of meditation, each with its own unique benefits for promoting health and well-being. When it comes to weight loss, mindfulness meditation, loving-kindness meditation, transcendental meditation, yoga, and body scan meditation are all effective options. By incorporating these practices into our daily routine, we can reduce stress, improve our relationship with food, and promote overall health, which can contribute to healthy weight loss.

Left blank intentionally

CHAPTER SIX

Mindful Eating: How to Incorporate Meditation into Your Eating Habits

Mindful eating is a practice that involves paying attention to your food and your eating habits. It can help you develop a better relationship with food and make healthier choices. Mindful eating can be a useful tool for weight loss, as it helps you become more aware of your body's hunger and fullness signals, which can prevent overeating.

Meditation is a powerful tool that can be used to enhance mindful eating. By practicing meditation regularly, you can develop a greater sense of awareness and become more mindful of your eating habits. In this article, we'll explore how to incorporate meditation into your eating habits and improve your relationship with food.

What is Mindful Eating?

Mindful eating is a practice that involves paying attention to your food and your eating habits. It's about being fully present in the moment while you eat, rather than eating mindlessly while distracted by other things. When you eat mindfully, you focus on the taste, texture, and smell of your food, as well as your body's hunger and fullness signals.

Mindful eating can help you develop a better relationship with food and make healthier choices. It can also help you lose weight, as it can prevent overeating and emotional eating.

How to Practice Mindful Eating

To practice mindful eating, start by taking a few deep breaths and bringing your attention to your body. Notice any sensations you're feeling, such as hunger or fullness, and use these signals to guide your eating.

When you sit down to eat, take a moment to appreciate your food. Notice the colors, textures, and smells of your meal. Take a bite and chew slowly, savoring the taste and texture of the food. Put down your fork or spoon between bites and take a moment to breathe and check in with your body.

Try to avoid distractions while you eat, such as watching TV or scrolling through your phone. Instead, focus on your food and your body. If your mind starts to wander, gently bring it back to the present moment.

Incorporating Meditation into Your Eating Habits

Meditation can be a powerful tool for enhancing mindful eating. By practicing meditation regularly, you can develop a greater sense of awareness and become more mindful of your eating habits.

Here are some tips for incorporating meditation into your eating habits:

1. **Meditate before you eat**

Take a few minutes to meditate before you sit down to eat. This can help you become more present and mindful of your eating habits. Focus on your breath and bring your attention to the present moment.

2. **Practice gratitude**

Take a moment to express gratitude for your food before you eat. This can help you develop a deeper appreciation for your meals and become more mindful of what you're eating.

3. **Use a mindful eating meditation**

There are many guided meditations available that can help you become more mindful of your eating habits. Look for a meditation that focuses on mindful eating, and try incorporating it into your daily routine.

4. Practice mindful breathing

During your meal, take a few deep breaths and focus on your breath. This can help you become more present and mindful of your eating habits.

5. Eat slowly and savor your food

Take your time when you eat and savor each bite. Notice the taste and texture of your food, and enjoy the experience of eating.

The Benefits of Mindful Eating

Incorporating meditation into your eating habits can have numerous benefits for your overall health and well-being. Here are some of the ways that mindful eating can benefit your body and mind:

1. **It can help you lose weight:** Mindful eating can prevent overeating and emotional eating, which can help you lose weight and maintain a healthy weight.

2. **It can improve your digestion:** Eating mindfully can improve your digestion by helping you chew your

CHAPTER SESVEN

Meditation and Physical Activity: Combining Meditation with Exercise for Weight Loss

Meditation has numerous benefits for physical and mental health, including weight loss. Combining meditation with physical activity is an effective strategy for those seeking to lose weight. The practice of meditation can help individuals develop a more mindful approach to physical activity, which can lead to increased motivation and adherence to an exercise routine.

One of the ways that meditation can support physical activity is by reducing stress and anxiety levels. Chronic stress can lead to weight gain due to the release of cortisol, a hormone that can increase appetite and promote fat storage. By reducing stress levels through regular meditation, individuals may be less likely to turn to food for comfort and may find it easier to make healthy choices.

Additionally, meditation can help individuals develop a greater sense of body awareness. By focusing on the present moment and paying attention to bodily sensations during exercise, individuals can develop a deeper connection to their bodies and better understand their physical needs. This can help individuals make more informed decisions about the type and duration of physical activity that is best for their body.

Meditation can also help individuals develop a positive mindset around physical activity. Rather than seeing exercise as a chore or punishment, individuals may begin to view it as a form of self-care and a way to nurture their body. This shift in mindset can lead to increased enjoyment of physical activity and may even result in individuals seeking out new forms of exercise that they find fulfilling.

Incorporating meditation into physical activity does not have to be complicated or time-consuming. Simple mindfulness techniques, such as focusing on the breath or paying attention to bodily sensations, can be practiced while engaging in a variety of physical activities. Walking meditation, for example, involves walking slowly and deliberately while focusing on the sensations of the feet on the ground and the movement of the body.

Other activities that can be paired with meditation include yoga, Pilates, and tai chi. These activities all focus on the connection between the mind and body and can be easily combined with mindfulness practices. By incorporating meditation into physical activity, individuals may find it easier to stick to a regular exercise routine and may experience greater benefits for their physical and mental health.

Overall, the combination of meditation and physical activity can be a powerful tool for weight loss and overall well-being. By reducing stress levels, increasing body awareness, and developing a positive mindset around physical activity, individuals can make sustainable changes to their health and achieve their weight loss goals.

CHAPTER EIGHT

Meditation for Emotional Eating: How to Manage Emotional Eating through Meditation

Meditation is an ancient practice that has been used to calm the mind, reduce stress, and promote well-being. In recent years, it has been shown that meditation can be an effective tool for weight loss. One area where meditation can be particularly helpful is in managing emotional eating.

Emotional eating is a common problem for many people. It is when someone eats not because they are physically hungry, but because they are experiencing emotions such as stress, anxiety, or sadness. Emotional eating can lead to overeating and weight gain, which can be difficult to reverse. However, with the help of meditation, it is possible to manage emotional eating and maintain a healthy weight.

Meditation helps to calm the mind and reduce stress, which can help to reduce the urge to eat in response to emotions. When you meditate, you are able to observe your thoughts and emotions without becoming overwhelmed by them.

This can help you to identify the root cause of your emotional eating and develop strategies to manage it.

There are several ways to use meditation to manage emotional eating. One approach is to use mindfulness meditation. This involves paying attention to the present moment without judgment. When you are mindful, you are aware of your thoughts and emotions without reacting to them. This can help you to observe your emotional eating patterns and develop strategies to manage them.

Another approach is to use guided meditations specifically designed to manage emotional eating. These meditations are often focused on building self-compassion and self-awareness. They may also include visualization exercises that help you to imagine a different response to your emotions. For example, instead of reaching for a cookie when you are feeling stressed, you might visualize going for a walk or taking a bath.

Meditation can also be combined with other practices, such as journaling, to help manage emotional eating. Writing down your thoughts and feelings can help you to identify patterns and triggers that lead to emotional eating. You can then use meditation to develop strategies to manage these triggers.

In addition to managing emotional eating, meditation can also help with overall weight loss. It has been shown to reduce stress, which can lead to a decrease in cortisol levels. Cortisol is a hormone that is released in response to stress, and high levels of cortisol have been linked to weight gain. By reducing stress and cortisol levels, meditation can help to promote weight loss.

Meditation can also help with mindful eating. When you are mindful, you are more aware of your body's hunger and fullness signals. This can help you to eat when you are physically hungry, rather than in response to emotions or external cues. By eating mindfully, you are more likely to make healthier food choices and eat in moderation.

Overall, meditation can be an effective tool for managing emotional eating and promoting weight loss. It helps to reduce stress, increase self-awareness, and promote mindfulness. By incorporating meditation into your daily routine, you can develop a healthier relationship with food and maintain a healthy weight.

CHAPTER NINE

Meditation for Cravings: How to Manage Food Cravings through Meditation

Meditation is a powerful tool that can be used to manage food cravings. Cravings are a natural part of the human experience, and they can be difficult to resist. However, with meditation, it is possible to train the mind to let go of these cravings and make healthier choices.

Cravings are often the result of stress or negative emotions. When we are stressed, our bodies produce cortisol, a hormone that can increase appetite and make us crave unhealthy foods. Negative emotions can also trigger cravings as a way of coping with difficult feelings. However, by practicing meditation, we can learn to manage stress and negative emotions in a healthier way.

One of the most effective ways to manage food cravings through meditation is to practice mindfulness. Mindfulness is the practice of being present and aware in the moment. By being mindful of our thoughts and feelings, we can become more aware of our cravings and learn to let them go.

To begin, find a quiet place where you can sit comfortably. Close your eyes and take a few deep breaths, focusing on your breath as it enters and leaves your body. As you breathe, become aware of any thoughts or feelings that arise. Don't judge these thoughts or try to push them away. Simply observe them and let them go.

As you become more comfortable with mindfulness meditation, you can begin to apply this practice to your eating habits. Before you eat, take a few deep breaths and focus on the food in front of you. Notice the colors, textures, and smells of the food. As you eat, savor each bite and be mindful of the sensations in your mouth. If you notice any cravings arising, simply observe them without judgment and let them go.

Another effective technique for managing food cravings through meditation is visualization. Visualization is the practice of creating a mental image of a desired outcome. By visualizing ourselves making healthy food choices and resisting cravings, we can train our minds to make healthier choices in real life.

To begin, find a quiet place where you can sit comfortably. Close your eyes and take a few deep breaths, focusing on your breath as it enters and leaves your body. As you breathe, visualize yourself making healthy food choices and resisting cravings. See yourself eating healthy foods that nourish your body and make you feel good. Visualize yourself feeling satisfied and happy with your choices.

As you become more comfortable with visualization, you can begin to use this technique in real-life situations. When a craving arises, take a few deep breaths and visualize yourself making a healthy choice. See yourself choosing a healthy snack or drink, and feel the satisfaction that comes with making a good choice.

In addition to mindfulness and visualization, there are many other meditation techniques that can be used to manage food cravings. For example, loving-kindness meditation involves sending love and compassion to ourselves and others. By practicing loving-kindness meditation, we can cultivate a sense of self-acceptance and self-love, which can help us resist the urge to indulge in unhealthy foods.

In conclusion, meditation is a powerful tool that can be used to manage food cravings and make healthier choices. By practicing mindfulness, visualization, and other meditation techniques, we can learn to manage stress and negative emotions in a healthier way, and train our minds to make healthier choices. With patience and practice, meditation can be a valuable tool for anyone looking to manage food cravings and make lasting changes to their eating habits.

CHAPTER TEN

Meditation and Body Image: How to Use Meditation to Improve Body Image and Self-Esteem

Meditation has been found to have numerous benefits for overall health and well-being, and one of the areas where it can be particularly helpful is in improving body image and self-esteem. Many people struggle with negative thoughts and feelings about their bodies, and this can have a significant impact on their mental health and quality of life. Fortunately, meditation can be a powerful tool for cultivating a more positive relationship with the body.

One of the ways in which meditation can help with body image is by promoting self-awareness and mindfulness. By becoming more aware of the thoughts and emotions that arise around body image, individuals can begin to identify patterns and triggers that may be contributing to negative self-talk and feelings of inadequacy. This increased awareness can then be used to develop more compassionate and positive attitudes towards the body.

Another benefit of meditation for body image is its ability to promote relaxation and reduce stress. Stress and anxiety can often exacerbate negative thoughts and feelings about the body, and can even contribute to the development of disordered eating behaviors. Meditation has been found to be an effective way to reduce stress and promote relaxation, which can in turn help individuals develop a more positive relationship with their bodies.

One specific type of meditation that has been found to be particularly helpful for body image is loving-kindness meditation. This practice involves cultivating feelings of warmth, kindness, and compassion towards oneself and others. By directing these positive feelings towards the body, individuals can begin to develop a more positive and accepting attitude towards their physical selves.

Body scan meditation is another form of mindfulness meditation that can be helpful for improving body image. This practice involves bringing awareness to different parts of the body and observing sensations without judgment. By focusing on the physical sensations of the body rather than judgments about appearance, individuals can develop a more grounded and accepting relationship with their bodies.

Meditation can also be a helpful tool for developing a more realistic and balanced perspective on the body. In a culture that often places a premium on thinness and physical perfection, it can be easy to develop unrealistic expectations and negative self-talk. By cultivating a more mindful and compassionate attitude towards the body, individuals can begin to develop a more realistic and balanced perspective on their physical selves.

In addition to these specific practices, incorporating mindfulness into daily life can also be helpful for improving body image. This can involve taking time to focus on the physical sensations of the body during everyday activities such as walking or showering, or simply taking a few deep breaths to center oneself and cultivate a sense of calm and roundedness.

In summary, meditation can be a powerful tool for improving body image and developing a more positive relationship with the body. By cultivating self-awareness, reducing stress and anxiety, and promoting self-compassion, individuals can begin to develop a more grounded and accepting attitude towards their physical selves. Whether through specific meditation practices or through mindfulness in daily life, incorporating meditation into one's routine can be a valuable step towards improving body image and self-esteem.

Left blank intentionally

CHAPTER ELEVEN

Meditation and Sleep: How to Use Meditation to Improve Sleep Quality for Better Weight Loss Results

Meditation is a well-known practice that has been used for centuries to achieve inner peace and improve overall well-being. Recently, there has been growing interest in the connection between meditation and weight loss. One aspect of this connection is the role that meditation can play in improving sleep quality, which in turn can lead to better weight loss results.

Sleep is an essential component of overall health and well-being, and it is well established that poor sleep quality can have negative effects on both physical and mental health. Additionally, research has shown that sleep deprivation can contribute to weight gain and obesity.

One way that meditation can help improve sleep quality is by reducing stress and anxiety. Stress and anxiety can disrupt sleep patterns and make it difficult to fall asleep or stay asleep throughout the night. Meditation has been shown to decrease levels of the stress hormone cortisol, which can help reduce feelings of stress and anxiety and promote relaxation.

Meditation can also help improve sleep quality by promoting relaxation and reducing tension in the body. Practicing meditation before bedtime can help calm the mind and prepare the body for sleep. Additionally, mindfulness meditation techniques can help individuals become more aware of physical sensations and reduce muscle tension, which can help promote deeper, more restful sleep.

Research has also shown that meditation can help regulate the circadian rhythm, the body's internal clock that regulates sleep-wake cycles. A regular meditation practice can help synchronize the circadian rhythm, leading to improved sleep quality and a more consistent sleep schedule.

Improved sleep quality can lead to better weight loss results in several ways. First, poor sleep quality can disrupt hormone levels, including those that regulate appetite and metabolism. Research has shown that sleep deprivation can lead to increased levels of the hunger hormone ghrelin and decreased levels of the satiety hormone leptin, which can lead to overeating and weight gain.

Second, poor sleep quality can lead to increased stress levels, which can contribute to overeating and unhealthy food choices. When we are stressed, our bodies release cortisol, which can increase appetite and lead to cravings for high-calorie, high-fat foods.

Finally, poor sleep quality can lead to fatigue and decreased motivation to engage in physical activity, which is essential for weight loss. When we are tired, we are less likely to exercise and more likely to choose sedentary activities, such as watching television or browsing social media.

By improving sleep quality through meditation, individuals can improve their overall health and well-being and potentially achieve better weight loss results. Incorporating meditation into a daily routine can be a simple and effective way to promote better sleep and support weight loss goals.

CHAPTER TWELVE

Meditation and Stress: How to Use Meditation to Manage Stress for Improved Weight Loss

Meditation has been found to have numerous benefits for physical and mental health, including its ability to help people manage stress. When it comes to weight loss, stress management is crucial as high levels of stress can lead to overeating and weight gain. In this article, we will explore the connection between meditation and stress, and how incorporating meditation into your weight loss journey can help you manage stress for improved results.

Stress and Weight Gain

Stress is a natural part of life, and it is normal to experience stress from time to time. However, chronic stress can have a negative impact on the body and lead to a range of health issues, including weight gain. When you are stressed, your body produces cortisol, a hormone that increases appetite and signals the body to store fat, particularly in the abdominal area. This can lead to weight gain, especially if you are already consuming more calories than you need.

In addition to the direct impact on weight gain, stress can also lead to emotional eating. Many people turn to food when they are stressed, as it provides comfort and can help distract from negative emotions. Unfortunately, emotional eating often leads to overeating and can contribute to weight gain.

How Meditation Can Help

Meditation has been found to be an effective tool for managing stress, as it can help to reduce cortisol levels and promote relaxation. When you meditate, you focus your attention on your breath, which helps to calm the mind and reduce feelings of anxiety and stress.

In addition to reducing cortisol levels, meditation has also been found to lower blood pressure and reduce inflammation in the body, both of which can be triggered by chronic stress.

Meditation Techniques for Stress Management

If you are new to meditation, there are a variety of techniques that you can try to help manage stress. Here are a few popular techniques:

1. **Mindfulness Meditation:** This technique involves focusing your attention on the present moment and accepting your thoughts and feelings without judgment.

2. **Loving-Kindness Meditation:** This technique involves cultivating feelings of love and compassion for yourself and others, which can help to reduce feelings of stress and negativity.

3. **Body Scan Meditation:** This technique involves focusing your attention on different parts of your body, starting at the toes and working your way up to the top of your head. This can help to promote relaxation and reduce feelings of tension in the body.

Incorporating Meditation into Your Weight Loss Journey

If you are looking to incorporate meditation into your weight loss journey, there are a few ways that you can do so. Here are some tips:

1. **Start Small:** If you are new to meditation, start with just a few minutes each day and gradually increase the amount of time that you spend meditating.

2. **Find a Quiet Place:** It can be helpful to find a quiet place where you can meditate without distraction. This could be a spare room in your house, a park, or any other place where you feel calm and relaxed.

3. **Use Guided Meditations:** There are many guided meditations available online that can help to guide you through the process of meditation. This can be helpful if you are new to meditation or if you are struggling to stay focused.

4. **Meditate Before Bed:** Meditating before bed can be particularly helpful for managing stress and improving sleep quality. This can also be a good time to reflect on your day and set intentions for the next day.

Conclusion

Incorporating meditation into your weight loss journey can be a powerful tool for managing stress and improving overall well-being. By reducing cortisol levels and promoting relaxation, meditation can help to reduce the negative impact of stress on the body and prevent overeating and weight gain. With a variety of meditation techniques to choose from and a few simple tips for incorporating meditation into your daily routine, it is easy to manage weight.

CHAPTER THIRTEEN

Overcoming Plateaus: How Meditation Can Help Break through Weight Loss Plateaus

Overcoming Plateaus: How Meditation Can Help Break through Weight Loss Plateaus

Weight loss plateaus are a common occurrence for many people who are trying to lose weight. Despite their best efforts, the scale may stop moving, and they may become frustrated with their progress. A weight loss plateau can occur for a variety of reasons, including a decrease in metabolism, hormonal changes, and a decrease in physical activity. Whatever the cause may be, it can be challenging to overcome a plateau and continue making progress towards your weight loss goals.

Meditation has been shown to be an effective tool for breaking through weight loss plateaus. It can help individuals stay focused on their goals, improve their mental well-being, and reduce stress, which can all contribute to weight loss success.

In this article, we'll explore the connection between meditation and breaking through weight loss plateaus.

What is a Weight Loss Plateau?

A weight loss plateau is a period where an individual stop losing weight despite continuing their weight loss efforts. It can be a frustrating experience, especially for those who have been making steady progress towards their weight loss goals.

Weight loss plateaus can occur for several reasons. For example, if you've been eating a low-calorie diet for an extended period, your body may adjust to the reduced calorie intake by slowing down your metabolism. As a result, you may stop losing weight, even if you continue to eat the same number of calories.

Another reason for a weight loss plateau could be hormonal changes. Women, in particular, may experience weight fluctuations due to hormonal changes during their menstrual cycle. These changes can cause water retention, leading to an increase in weight.

Additionally, a decrease in physical activity can also cause a weight loss plateau. If you've been exercising regularly and then suddenly stop, your body may adjust to the decreased activity level, leading to a decrease in metabolism and a plateau in weight loss.

How Meditation Can Help Overcome Plateaus

Meditation can be an effective tool for breaking through weight loss plateaus. Here are some ways meditation can help:

1. Mindful Eating

Meditation can help individuals become more aware of their eating habits and make more conscious food choices. By practicing mindfulness while eating, you can learn to pay attention to your hunger and fullness cues and avoid overeating. Overeating can lead to weight gain, and by learning to control your food intake, you can break through a weight loss plateau.

2. Stress Reduction

Stress is a common cause of weight gain and can contribute to weight loss plateaus. Stress can lead to overeating, poor food choices, and decreased physical activity, all of which can hinder weight loss progress. Meditation can help reduce stress levels and promote a sense of calm and relaxation. By reducing stress, individuals may be more likely to make healthier food choices and engage in regular physical activity, leading to weight loss success.

3. Improved Sleep Quality

Lack of sleep has been linked to weight gain and can contribute to weight loss plateaus. Poor sleep can affect hormones that regulate hunger and appetite, leading to overeating and weight gain. Meditation has been shown to improve sleep quality and promote relaxation, which can contribute to weight loss success.

4. Motivation and Focus

Meditation can help individuals stay motivated and focused on their weight loss goals. By practicing mindfulness, individuals can develop a sense of purpose and direction, leading to increased motivation to make healthy lifestyle changes. By staying focused on their goals, individuals can overcome weight loss plateaus and continue to make progress towards their weight loss goals.

Conclusion

Breaking through a weight loss plateau can be a challenging experience. However, incorporating meditation into your weight loss journey can be an effective tool for overcoming plateaus and achieving weight loss success. By practicing mindfulness and reducing stress levels, individuals can make healthier food.

CHAPTER FORTEEN

Meditation and Social Support: How to Use Group Meditation to Boost Motivation and Accountability

Meditation is often thought of as a solitary practice, but it can also be a powerful tool for building social support and accountability. Group meditation sessions can help individuals build a sense of community and connectedness, which can in turn boost motivation and help with weight loss goals.

There are several ways in which group meditation can be used to support weight loss efforts. First, simply being part of a group can provide a sense of accountability. Knowing that others are counting on you to show up and participate can help you stay committed to your goals. This can be especially important during times when motivation is low or when you are struggling to stay on track.

In addition to accountability, group meditation can also provide a sense of social support. When you meditate with others, you may feel a sense of camaraderie and shared purpose. This can help to combat feelings of isolation or loneliness that may arise when working on weight loss goals.

There are several ways to find group meditation opportunities. Some yoga studios, meditation centers, and community centers offer regular group meditation sessions. You may also be able to find online communities or virtual meditation groups that can provide social support and accountability.

When participating in a group meditation session, it is important to set clear intentions and goals for your practice. This can help to ensure that you are focusing on the areas of your life that are most important to you. For example, you may choose to set an intention to cultivate self-compassion or to focus on gratitude. You may also choose to use visualization or other techniques to help you stay motivated and focused on your weight loss goals.

In addition to group meditation sessions, there are other ways to build social support and accountability into your weight loss efforts. For example, you may choose to join a weight loss support group or to work with a personal trainer or coach. These types of support can provide additional motivation and accountability, which can be especially helpful during times of difficulty or when faced with obstacles.

Ultimately, the key to using meditation and social support for weight loss is to stay committed to your goals and to seek out the resources and support that will help you achieve them. By building a strong support network and committing to a regular meditation practice, you can stay focused and motivated on your weight loss journey.

CHAPTER FIFTEEN

Meditation for Binge Eating Disorder: How Meditation Can Help Manage Binge Eating

Meditation has been proven to be a powerful tool for managing various eating disorders, including binge eating disorder (BED). Binge eating disorder is characterized by recurrent episodes of consuming large amounts of food in a short period, accompanied by a feeling of loss of control. These episodes can be distressing and can have significant physical and emotional consequences. Incorporating meditation into the treatment plan for binge eating disorder can help individuals manage their symptoms and develop a healthier relationship with food and their bodies.

Mindful Eating

One of the primary ways in which meditation can help with binge eating disorder is through mindful eating. Mindful eating is a practice that involves paying attention to the present moment and the experience of eating without judgment. It encourages individuals to tune into their body's hunger and fullness cues, as well as to explore their thoughts, emotions, and sensations around food.

By practicing mindful eating, individuals with binge eating disorder can become more aware of their triggers, such as emotional stress or boredom, and their body's physical cues. This awareness allows them to differentiate between physical hunger and emotional hunger, helping them make conscious choices about when and what to eat.

Meditation Techniques for Binge Eating Disorder

Several meditation techniques can be beneficial for managing binge eating disorder. Here are a few:

1. **Body Scan Meditation:** This technique involves systematically focusing on each part of the body, noticing any sensations or tension. It helps individuals develop a deeper connection with their bodies and increase body awareness, which can aid in recognizing physical hunger and fullness cues.

2. **Loving-Kindness Meditation:** This practice involves cultivating feelings of love, compassion, and kindness toward oneself and others. For individuals with binge eating disorder, it can help develop self-

acceptance and self-compassion, reducing negative self-talk and judgment surrounding food and eating habits.

3. **Breathing Meditation:** Focusing on the breath is a common meditation technique that can help individuals ground themselves in the present moment and reduce stress and anxiety, which are often triggers for binge eating episodes.

4. **Managing Emotions and Stress**

Binge eating disorder is often associated with emotional distress and stress. Many individuals turn to food as a way to cope with difficult emotions or to numb their feelings temporarily. Meditation can be a powerful tool for managing emotions and reducing stress, which, in turn, can help individuals reduce the frequency and intensity of binge eating episodes.

Regular meditation practice can help individuals develop skills to identify and regulate their emotions effectively. By cultivating mindfulness, individuals can observe their emotions without judgment, allowing them to respond rather than react impulsively. This increased self-awareness can lead to more adaptive coping mechanisms and a reduction in emotional eating behaviors.

Reducing Anxiety and Depression

Anxiety and depression often co-occur with binge eating disorder. Meditation has been shown to reduce symptoms of anxiety and depression by calming the mind and promoting a sense of inner peace and well-being. By incorporating meditation into the treatment plan, individuals with binge eating disorder can find relief from the emotional turmoil that often fuels their disordered eating patterns.

Building a Supportive Mindset

Meditation can also help individuals with binge eating disorder build a supportive mindset towards themselves and their bodies. Through meditation, individuals can cultivate self-compassion, self-acceptance, and a positive body image. This shift in mindset can foster a healthier relationship with food and a more balanced approach to eating.

Incorporating Meditation into Treatment

To incorporate meditation into the treatment of binge eating disorder, it is important to work with a qualified healthcare professional or therapist who specializes in eating disorders. They can guide you through the process, provide support, and tailor the meditation practices to your specific needs and challenges.

In addition to formal meditation sessions, integrating mindfulness into daily life can be beneficial. This can involve taking a few mindful breaths before meals, practicing mindful walking, or engaging in other activities with full presence and awareness.

It is essential to remember that meditation is not a standalone treatment for binge eating disorder but rather a complementary practice that can enhance the effectiveness of a comprehensive treatment plan. It is crucial to seek professional help, including therapy, nutritional guidance, and support groups, to address the underlying psychological and emotional factors contributing to binge eating disorder.

In conclusion, meditation can be a valuable tool for individuals with binge eating disorder in managing their condition. By cultivating mindfulness, emotional regulation, and self-compassion, meditation can help individuals develop a healthier relationship with food and manage binge eating behaviors more effectively. It is important to approach meditation as part of a comprehensive treatment plan that includes therapy and other forms of support. With dedication and practice, individuals can find greater peace.

Left blank intentionally

CHAPTER SIXTEEN

Meditation and Self-Care: How to Use Meditation to Prioritize Self-Care for Better Weight Loss Results

Meditation is not only a powerful tool for stress reduction and mindfulness but can also be an effective practice for prioritizing self-care, which is essential for achieving better weight loss results. Self-care involves taking deliberate actions to nurture and prioritize your physical, mental, and emotional well-being. By incorporating meditation into your self-care routine, you can enhance your weight loss journey and improve your overall health and happiness.

1. **Developing Self-Awareness:** Meditation allows you to cultivate self-awareness by paying attention to your thoughts, emotions, and bodily sensations. This awareness helps you recognize and understand your personal needs and triggers. By being aware of your body's signals, you can make conscious decisions about your nutrition, exercise, and overall well-being. This self-awareness supports healthier

choices and helps you avoid mindless eating or neglecting your self-care routines.

2. **Stress Reduction:** Chronic stress can hinder weight loss progress by affecting your hormones, appetite, and cravings. Incorporating meditation into your self-care routine can help reduce stress levels by activating the relaxation response. Meditation encourages deep breathing, relaxation, and the release of tension in the body. By managing stress through regular meditation practice, you create a more supportive environment for weight loss and overall well-being.

3. **Emotional Balance:** Emotional eating can sabotage weight loss efforts. Meditation can help you cultivate emotional balance and resilience by providing a safe space to explore and process your emotions. By practicing mindfulness, you develop a non-judgmental attitude toward your emotions, allowing them to arise and pass without attaching to them. This emotional awareness enables you to respond to emotional triggers with greater clarity

and make healthier choices for nourishing your body.

4. **Enhancing Body-Mind Connection:** Meditation strengthens the connection between your mind and body, allowing you to listen to your body's signals and respond accordingly. This awareness helps you tune into your hunger and fullness cues, distinguishing between physical and emotional hunger. By mindfully eating, you can savor and enjoy your meals, eating until you are satisfied rather than overindulging. This mindful approach to eating supports healthier portion control and more balanced food choices.

5. **Cultivating Self-Compassion:** Weight loss journeys can be challenging and sometimes accompanied by self-criticism and negative self-talk. Meditation fosters self-compassion, a vital aspect of self-care. Through meditation, you learn to treat yourself with kindness, understanding, and acceptance. By being compassionate toward yourself, you can better navigate setbacks, overcome obstacles, and maintain motivation throughout your weight loss journey.

6. **Prioritizing Rest and Recovery:** Adequate rest and recovery are essential for weight loss and overall well-being. Incorporating meditation into your self-care routine can help you prioritize and enhance your sleep quality. Meditation promotes relaxation and reduces racing thoughts, enabling you to unwind and prepare for restful sleep. Better sleep supports optimal metabolism, hormone regulation, and energy levels, which are crucial for successful weight loss.

7. **Mindful Movement:** In addition to meditation, integrating mindful movement practices into your self-care routine can further support weight loss. Activities like yoga, tai chi, or walking meditation combine movement and mindfulness, fostering a deeper connection with your body and promoting physical well-being. These practices can improve flexibility, strength, and body awareness, complementing your weight loss efforts.

8. **Setting Boundaries and Saying No:** Self-care involves setting boundaries and prioritizing your needs. Through meditation, you develop a deeper sense of self and clarity about your values. This

awareness empowers you to say no to activities, commitments, or relationships that do not align with your well-being or weight loss goals. By setting boundaries and honoring your needs, you create space for self-care practices that support your overall health and weight loss journey.

9. **Mindful Stress Management:** Weight loss journeys can be accompanied by various stressors, including social pressures, time constraints, and personal expectations. Meditation can help you develop effective stress management strategies. By practicing mindfulness, you can observe your stress triggers and respond to them with greater awareness and resilience. This reduces the likelihood of turning to food as a coping mechanism and supports healthier stress management techniques.

10. **Nurturing Your Mind and Spirit:** Self-care extends beyond physical well-being. It involves nourishing your mind and spirit through activities that bring joy, inspiration, and personal growth. Meditation provides a platform for introspection, creativity, and connecting with your inner self. By incorporating

meditation into your self-care routine, you create space for reflection, gratitude, and self-expression, enhancing your overall well-being and supporting your weight loss goals.

Incorporating meditation into your self-care routine is a powerful way to prioritize your well-being and enhance your weight loss journey. By cultivating self-awareness, managing stress, fostering emotional balance, and nurturing your mind and body, you create a supportive environment for successful weight loss and overall health. Remember that self-care is a continuous practice, and with dedication and mindfulness, you can transform your relationship with yourself and achieve long-lasting weight loss results.

CHAPTER SEVENTEEN

Meditation and Mindset: How to Use Meditation to Shift Your Mindset for Successful Weight Loss

When it comes to weight loss, cultivating the right mindset is crucial for long-term success. Our mindset influences our thoughts, beliefs, and behaviors, shaping the choices we make regarding our health and well-being. Meditation can be a powerful tool for shifting our mindset and creating a positive and empowered mindset that supports successful weight loss. By incorporating meditation into your routine, you can transform your relationship with your body, food, and exercise, setting the stage for lasting change.

1. **Developing Self-Awareness:** Meditation helps us develop self-awareness by bringing our attention to the present moment. Through regular practice, we become more attuned to our thoughts, emotions, and physical sensations. This self-awareness is essential for recognizing and challenging negative or limiting beliefs about our bodies and weight loss. By becoming aware of these thoughts, we can replace them with more positive and empowering ones.

2. **Cultivating a Non-Judgmental Attitude:** Meditation encourages a non-judgmental attitude toward our thoughts and experiences. Instead of labeling thoughts as good or bad, right or wrong, we learn to observe them with curiosity and compassion. This attitude extends to our body and weight loss journey. By practicing non-judgment, we can let go of self-criticism and embrace self-acceptance, fostering a positive and supportive mindset.

3. **Challenging Limiting Beliefs:** Many individuals hold onto limiting beliefs about their ability to lose weight or maintain a healthy lifestyle. These beliefs can sabotage progress and create self-doubt. Through meditation, we can identify and challenge these beliefs. By creating a space for self-reflection and inquiry, we can explore the origins of these beliefs and replace them with empowering ones. Meditation helps us tap into our inner wisdom and recognize that we have the power to change our mindset and achieve our weight loss goals.

4. **Letting Go of Perfectionism:** Perfectionism can be a significant obstacle on the weight loss journey. It can lead to feelings of inadequacy, self-sabotage,

and an all-or-nothing mindset. Meditation teaches us to let go of perfectionism and embrace progress over perfection. By cultivating mindfulness and self-compassion, we can appreciate the small steps and improvements we make along the way. This mindset shift allows us to celebrate our successes and maintain motivation even when faced with setbacks.

5. **Embracing Self-Compassion:** Self-compassion is a fundamental aspect of a positive weight loss mindset. It involves treating ourselves with kindness, understanding, and acceptance, especially in moments of difficulty or failure. Meditation helps us cultivate self-compassion by fostering a sense of inner calm and nurturing self-talk. Through meditation, we learn to be gentle with ourselves, acknowledge our challenges, and respond to them with self-care and self-love.

6. **Focusing on the Present Moment:** Weight loss journeys can be overwhelming when we get caught up in the past or worry about the future. Meditation brings our attention back to the present moment, helping us let go of regrets or anxieties. By focusing

on the here and now, we can make conscious choices that align with our weight loss goals. This shift in mindset allows us to appreciate the journey and make empowered decisions in the present moment.

7. **Visualizing Success:** Meditation can be a powerful tool for visualizing success and reinforcing positive affirmations. By incorporating visualization techniques into your practice, you can imagine yourself reaching your weight loss goals, feeling healthy, confident, and vibrant. Visualization helps align your subconscious mind with your desired outcome, creating a positive and motivated mindset that supports your weight loss journey.

8. **Building Resilience:** Weight loss journeys often involve challenges and setbacks. Developing resilience is essential for maintaining motivation and bouncing back from difficulties. Meditation helps us build resilience by training our minds to stay present, focus on solutions, and maintain a positive outlook. By practicing meditation regularly, we strengthen our ability to navigate obstacles, stay

committed to our goals, and cultivate a resilient mindset.

9. **Cultivating Gratitude:** Gratitude is a powerful mindset shift that can transform our weight loss journey. Meditation allows us to cultivate gratitude by shifting our attention to the positive aspects of our lives. By focusing on what we are grateful for, we shift our mindset from scarcity to abundance. This mindset shift helps us appreciate our bodies, the progress we make, and the support systems that surround us.

10. **Nurturing a Growth Mindset:** A growth mindset is essential for successful weight loss. It involves embracing challenges, seeing setbacks as opportunities for growth, and believing in our ability to change. Meditation fosters a growth mindset by cultivating resilience, self-awareness, and a positive attitude toward change. By practicing meditation, we develop the mindset that our weight loss journey is a learning experience, and every step forward is a valuable lesson.

Incorporating meditation into your daily routine can have profound effects on your mindset and support successful weight loss. By developing self-awareness, challenging limiting beliefs, embracing self-compassion, and nurturing a positive and growth-oriented mindset, you can create the mental foundation necessary for sustainable weight loss. Remember that meditation is a practice, and consistency is key. Over time, you will experience the transformative power of meditation on your mindset and weight loss journey.

CHAPTER EIGHTEEN

Meditation and Cravings: How to Use Meditation to Manage Sugar Cravings

Sugar cravings can be a common challenge when trying to maintain a healthy diet or lose weight. These intense desires for sweet treats can often derail our progress and lead to overconsumption of sugary foods. However, incorporating meditation into your routine can be a powerful tool for managing sugar cravings and developing a healthier relationship with food. By practicing mindfulness and cultivating awareness, you can better understand the underlying causes of your cravings and respond to them in a more balanced and empowered way.

1. **Developing Mindful Awareness:** Meditation cultivates mindful awareness, which is the practice of observing our thoughts, emotions, and bodily sensations without judgment. By bringing mindful awareness to our sugar cravings, we can gain insight into their origin and nature. Instead of reacting impulsively to cravings, we can pause, take a deep breath, and observe our thoughts and bodily

sensations. This awareness helps us understand the triggers and patterns behind our cravings, allowing us to respond with intention and make healthier choices.

2. **Recognizing Emotional Cravings:** Sugar cravings are not always about physical hunger but can often be driven by emotions. Stress, boredom, loneliness, or sadness can trigger a desire for sugary foods as a way to seek comfort or distraction. Through meditation, we become more attuned to our emotional states and the ways in which we seek solace in food. By recognizing and acknowledging our emotions, we can address them directly through self-care activities or healthier coping mechanisms instead of relying on sugar for temporary relief.

3. **Cultivating Mindful Eating:** Mindful eating is a practice that involves paying full attention to the experience of eating. By bringing mindfulness to the act of consuming sugary foods, we can savor each bite, notice the flavors and textures, and fully enjoy the experience. This heightened awareness helps us develop a deeper sense of satisfaction from smaller portions, reducing the need for excessive sugar

intake. Meditation can support mindful eating by training us to be present in the moment, to listen to our bodies, and to eat in a way that nourishes us rather than being driven solely by cravings.

4. **Pausing and Reflecting:** Meditation teaches us the importance of pausing and reflecting before acting on our impulses. When a sugar craving arises, rather than immediately giving in to it, we can take a moment to pause, breathe, and reflect on our true needs. Is the craving a result of physical hunger, emotional distress, or habit? By giving ourselves this space to reflect, we can respond with greater awareness and choose healthier alternatives or strategies to address our underlying needs.

5. **Finding Inner Calm:** Cravings often come with a sense of urgency and restlessness. Meditation helps us find inner calm and peace amidst the cravings. By dedicating a few minutes each day to meditation, we can cultivate a sense of tranquility that allows us to observe cravings without feeling compelled to act upon them. This inner calm helps us detach from the intensity of the craving and make more conscious

decisions based on our long-term goals rather than momentary impulses.

6. **Practicing Urge Surfing:** Urge surfing is a technique often used in mindfulness-based approaches to manage cravings. It involves observing the ebb and flow of cravings without acting on them. Through meditation, we can develop the skills to ride out the waves of cravings, knowing that they will eventually subside. By recognizing that cravings are temporary sensations, we can build our capacity to tolerate discomfort and make healthier choices in the face of intense sugar cravings.

7. **Cultivating Gratitude for Health:** Meditation fosters a sense of gratitude and appreciation for the body and its well-being. By regularly practicing gratitude, we can shift our focus from the temporary pleasure of sugary foods to the long-term benefits of a healthy diet. Reflecting on the nourishment and vitality our bodies receive from wholesome foods can reduce the allure of sugar cravings and reinforce our commitment to making healthier choices.

8. **Using Mantras and Affirmations:** Meditation allows us to harness the power of positive affirmations and

mantras. By creating affirmations related to managing sugar cravings and repeating them during meditation, we can reprogram our subconscious mind and shift our beliefs around sugary foods. Affirmations like "I am in control of my cravings" or "I choose nourishing foods that support my well-being" can empower us to make healthier choices and reduce our reliance on sugar.

9. **Seeking Support:** Incorporating meditation into your journey of managing sugar cravings can be enhanced by seeking support from others. Joining a meditation group or finding a community of like-minded individuals can provide encouragement, accountability, and a space to share experiences and insights. Sharing your struggles and successes with others can strengthen your resolve and provide valuable perspectives and strategies for managing cravings.

10. **Patience and Persistence:** Managing sugar cravings through meditation is a gradual process that requires patience and persistence. Just as meditation is a practice that develops over time, so too is the ability to manage cravings. Be kind to

yourself and embrace the journey, knowing that each moment of mindfulness contributes to your overall progress. With continued practice and self-compassion, you can cultivate a healthier relationship with sugar and achieve greater balance in your diet.

Incorporating meditation into your routine can be a transformative approach to managing sugar cravings and supporting your weight loss goals. By developing mindful awareness, addressing emotional triggers, practicing mindful eating, and cultivating inner calm, you can navigate the challenges of sugar cravings with greater ease and make empowered choices that align with your long-term well-being. Remember that meditation is a personal journey, and finding the techniques and practices that resonate with you is key to harnessing its power in managing sugar cravings effectively.

CHAPTER NINETEEN

Meditation and Sustainable Weight Loss: How to Use Meditation to Maintain Weight Loss Results

Achieving sustainable weight loss involves not only reaching your desired weight but also maintaining it over the long term. This requires a holistic approach that addresses not only dietary and exercise habits but also the underlying psychological and emotional factors that influence our relationship with food and our bodies. Meditation can be a powerful tool for supporting sustainable weight loss by fostering self-awareness, cultivating a positive mindset, managing stress, and promoting mindful eating. By incorporating meditation into your weight loss journey, you can create a solid foundation for lasting success.

1. **Cultivating Self-Awareness:** Meditation is a practice of self-reflection and self-observation. Through regular meditation sessions, you develop the ability to tune in to your body's signals, emotions, and thoughts. This heightened self-awareness is essential for sustainable weight loss because it allows you to recognize and understand your

triggers, patterns, and behaviors related to food and exercise. By becoming more aware of your habits and tendencies, you can make conscious choices that align with your long-term health goals.

2. **Mindfulness for Eating:** Mindfulness is a key component of meditation and involves bringing non-judgmental awareness to the present moment. When applied to eating, mindfulness can transform your relationship with food. By practicing mindful eating, you can savor each bite, pay attention to hunger and fullness cues, and make conscious choices about what and how much you eat. This approach helps you develop a greater appreciation for the nourishment and pleasure that food provides, leading to more balanced and mindful eating habits.

3. **Managing Emotional Eating:** Emotional eating is a common challenge for many people, and it can hinder sustainable weight loss efforts. Meditation can help you develop the skills to manage emotional eating by cultivating emotional resilience and providing tools for self-soothing and stress management. By practicing meditation regularly,

you can enhance your ability to identify and cope with emotional triggers without turning to food for comfort or distraction.

4. **Developing a Positive Mindset:** A positive mindset is crucial for sustainable weight loss. Meditation can help you cultivate a positive and empowering mindset by training you to focus on the present moment, challenge negative self-talk, and embrace self-compassion. By practicing gratitude and positive affirmations during meditation, you can shift your mindset from a place of self-criticism and doubt to one of self-acceptance and belief in your ability to make healthy choices.

5. **Stress Management:** Stress is a significant contributor to weight gain and difficulty in maintaining weight loss. Meditation is a powerful stress management tool that activates the body's relaxation response and promotes a state of calm. By incorporating meditation into your daily routine, you can reduce stress levels, enhance resilience to stressors, and prevent stress-induced eating. This, in turn, supports sustainable weight loss by preventing emotional and stress-related overeating.

6. **Building Healthy Habits:** Sustainable weight loss is not about quick fixes or temporary changes but about establishing healthy habits that you can maintain for the long term. Meditation can help you develop the discipline, focus, and motivation needed to build and maintain healthy habits. By incorporating meditation into your routine, you strengthen your willpower, enhance your ability to stay consistent with exercise and dietary choices, and foster a greater sense of self-control.

7. **Body Acceptance and Self-Love:** Sustainable weight loss is not solely about reaching a specific number on the scale but also about cultivating a positive body image and practicing self-love. Meditation promotes body acceptance by helping you develop a compassionate and non-judgmental attitude toward your body. By cultivating self-love and embracing your body as it is, you can foster a healthy relationship with yourself and maintain weight loss from a place of self-care rather than self-criticism.

8. **Overcoming Plateaus and Challenges:** Weight loss journeys are often accompanied by plateaus and

challenges. Meditation can help you navigate these obstacles with greater ease and resilience. By practicing meditation, you develop mental flexibility, adaptability, and problem-solving skills. This allows you to approach plateaus and challenges with a calm and creative mindset, exploring new strategies and staying motivated even when progress may seem slow.

9. **Accountability and Support:** Meditation can be a solitary practice, but it can also be integrated into a community or support network. By joining meditation groups or seeking support from like-minded individuals, you can create a sense of accountability and shared experiences. Sharing your weight loss journey and meditation practice with others can provide encouragement, inspiration, and guidance, reinforcing your commitment to sustainable weight loss.

10. **Cultivating Balance:** Sustainable weight loss is not about extreme restrictions or deprivation but about finding balance and nourishing your body and mind. Meditation can help you cultivate a sense of balance by promoting self-awareness, mindfulness, and self-

compassion. By being attuned to your body's needs and honoring them with balanced choices, you can achieve sustainable weight loss while maintaining overall well-being.

Incorporating meditation into your weight loss journey can have profound effects on your ability to achieve and maintain sustainable weight loss. By cultivating self-awareness, practicing mindful eating, managing emotional eating, developing a positive mindset, managing stress, building healthy habits, fostering body acceptance, overcoming challenges, seeking support, and cultivating balance, you create a solid foundation for long-term success. Remember that meditation is a practice, and consistency is key. With dedication and patience, you can harness the power of meditation to support your weight loss goals and create a healthier and more fulfilling life

CHAPTER TWENTY

Conclusion: The Power of Meditation in Your Weight Loss Journey

In conclusion, the power of meditation in your weight loss journey cannot be overstated. It is a transformative practice that goes beyond the physical aspects of weight loss and addresses the underlying psychological and emotional factors that often contribute to weight gain and difficulty in sustaining weight loss. By incorporating meditation into your daily routine, you can cultivate self-awareness, enhance mindfulness, manage stress, develop a positive mindset, and build healthy habits that support long-term weight management.

Meditation provides a powerful tool for self-reflection and self-observation, allowing you to become more aware of your thoughts, emotions, and behaviors related to food and your body. This heightened self-awareness enables you to recognize and understand your triggers, patterns, and habits, empowering you to make conscious choices that align with your weight loss goals. It helps you tune in to your body's signals, such as hunger and fullness cues, and make mindful decisions about what and how much you eat.

One of the remarkable benefits of meditation is its ability to cultivate mindfulness. Mindful eating, in particular, helps you develop a deeper connection with your food, savor each bite, and make deliberate choices that nourish your body. By practicing mindfulness, you can break free from automatic eating habits, emotional eating, and mindless snacking, leading to more balanced and mindful eating patterns.

Stress is a common obstacle in weight loss journeys, as it often triggers emotional eating and disrupts healthy habits. Fortunately, meditation is an excellent tool for managing stress. It activates the body's relaxation response, reducing stress levels and promoting a sense of calm and inner peace. Through regular meditation practice, you can enhance your resilience to stress, improve emotional well-being, and prevent stress-induced eating.

A positive mindset is crucial for sustainable weight loss. Meditation helps you cultivate a positive and empowering mindset by training you to focus on the present moment, challenge negative self-talk, and cultivate self-compassion.

By practicing gratitude, positive affirmations, and visualization techniques during meditation, you can shift your mindset from self-doubt and self-criticism to self-acceptance and belief in your ability to achieve your weight loss goals.

Building healthy habits is essential for long-term weight management. Meditation can provide the discipline, focus, and motivation needed to establish and maintain healthy habits. It strengthens your willpower, enhances self-control, and fosters a sense of self-discipline that supports your weight loss efforts.

Furthermore, meditation promotes body acceptance and self-love. It helps you develop a compassionate and non-judgmental attitude toward your body, fostering a healthier relationship with yourself. By embracing your body as it is and practicing self-care, you can maintain weight loss from a place of self-acceptance rather than self-criticism.

Incorporating meditation into your weight loss journey is a personal and transformative process. It requires consistency, commitment, and patience. Remember that meditation is not a quick fix but a practice that unfolds over time. Embrace the journey, be gentle with yourself, and celebrate small victories along the way.

As you embark on your weight loss journey, consider integrating meditation into your daily routine. Explore different meditation techniques and find what resonates with you. Whether it's mindfulness meditation, loving-kindness meditation, or guided visualizations, find the practices that support your well-being and align with your goals.

The power of meditation lies in its ability to bring harmony and balance to your mind, body, and spirit. It empowers you to make conscious choices, manage stress, cultivate a positive mindset, and build healthy habits that contribute to sustainable weight loss. Embrace the transformative potential of meditation and allow it to guide you on your journey toward a healthier, happier, and more fulfilling life.